PROFILES

Edith Cavell
Nigel Richardson

Illustrated by
Edward Mortelmans

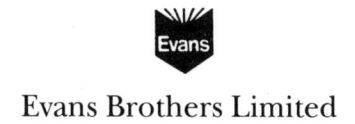

Evans Brothers Limited

Published by Evans Brothers Limited
2A Portman Mansions
Chiltern Street
London W1M 1LE

First published in Great Britain in 1985 by
Hamish Hamilton Children's Books

© Nigel Richardson (text) 1985

© Edward Mortelmans (illustrations) 1985

All Rights Reserved. No part of this publication may be reproduced, stored in a retrieval system or transmitted in any form or by any means, electronic, mechanical, photocopying, recording or otherwise, without prior permission of Evans Brothers Limited.

Reprinted 1987, 1994

Typeset by Pioneer

Printed by Qualitex Printing Limited
Tudor Street, Cardiff CF1 8UR,
Great Britain
Tel: (01222) 228088

ISBN 0 237 60020 X

Titles in this series

Ian Botham	0 237 60030 7	Gandhi	0 237 60011 0
Edith Cavell	0 237 60020 X	Indira Gandhi	0 237 60025 0
Marie Curie	0 237 60024 2	Bob Geldof	0 237 60031 5
Roald Dahl	0 237 60010 2	Amy Johnson	0 237 60032 3
Thomas Edison	0 237 60006 4	Helen Keller	0 237 60016 1
Alexander Fleming	0 237 60013 7	John F. Kennedy	0 237 60029 3
John Lennon	0 237 60021 8	Florence Nightingale	0 237 60018 8
Martin Luther King	0 237 60007 2	Emmeline Pankhurst	0 237 60019 6
Nelson Mandela	0 237 60026 9	Pope John Paul II	0 237 60005 6
Bob Marley	0 237 60017 X	Prince Philip	0 237 60012 9
Mother Teresa	0 237 60008 0	Princess of Wales	0 237 60023 4
Margot Fonteyn	0 237 60033 1	Queen Victoria	0 237 60001 3
Anne Frank	0 237 60015 3	Viv Richards	0 237 60027 7
Elizabeth Fry	0 237 60028 5	Margaret Thatcher	0 237 60003 X

Contents

1	COMING HOME	9
2	A NORFOLK CHILD	12
3	A LOVELY GIRL	16
4	THE LONDON HOSPITAL	22
5	THE RUE DE LA CULTURE	27
6	A LOYAL FRIEND	32
7	WAR	39
8	A HIGHER DUTY THAN PRUDENCE	42
9	I CANNOT EXPRESS ENOUGH THANKS	46
10	ARREST	50
11	THEY WANT MY LIFE	53
12	BRUSSELS: DAWN; OCTOBER 12th	56
13	THE SUPREME LESSON	59

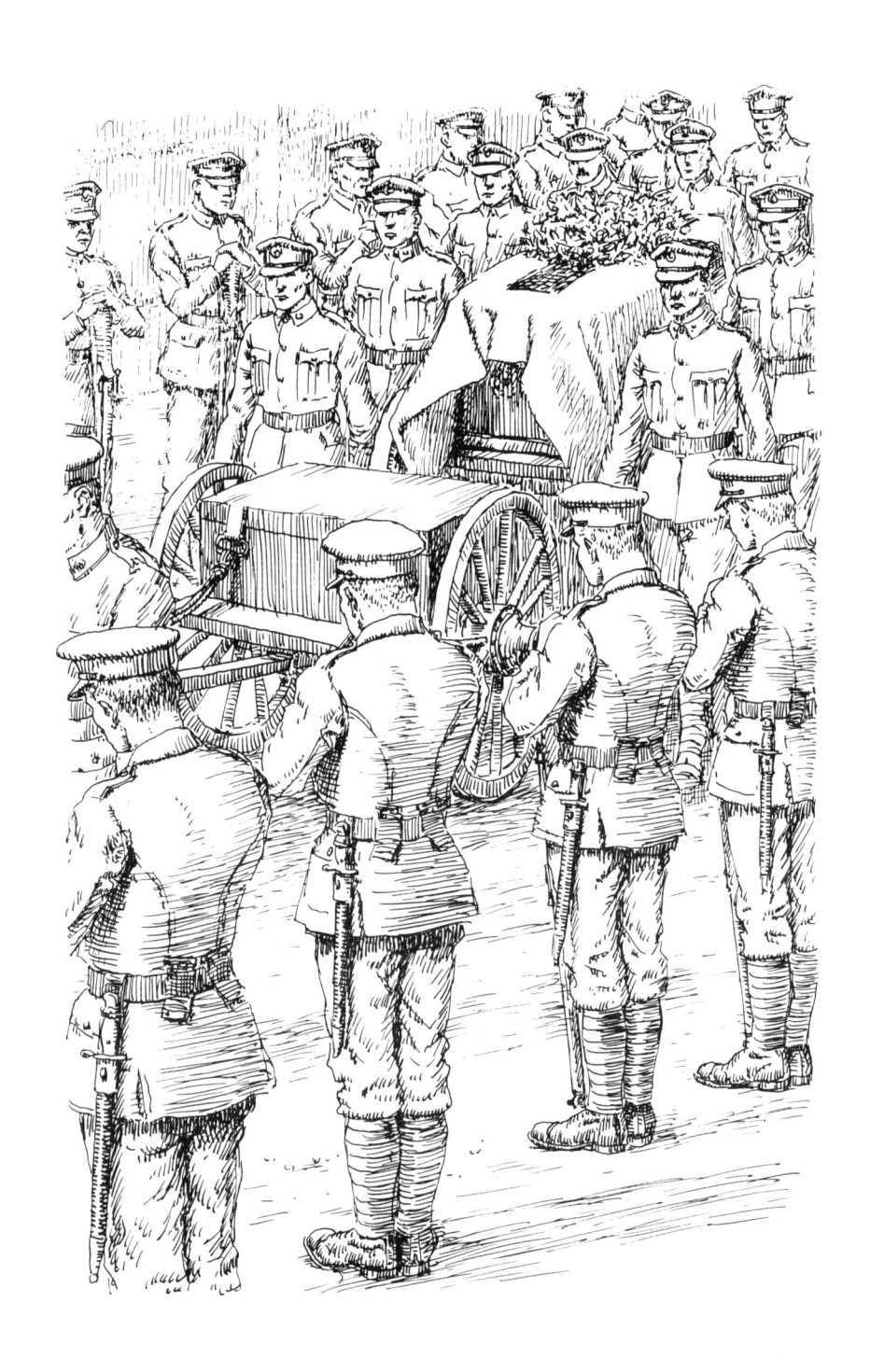

1 Coming Home

May 14th 1919. It was a beautiful sunny evening, but there was a strong east wind as the naval destroyer *Rowena* waited outside Dover harbour. Two small boats steamed towards the quay carrying a group of mourners, many wreaths of flowers — including one from the Queen of Belgium — and a single coffin. On the coffin lid were the words 'Edith Cavell. Born December 4th 1865. Died October 12th 1915.'

Fifteen minutes earlier a signal had gone out, and all the warships in the harbour had lowered their flags as a mark of respect. Now the coffin was taken ashore by sailors. Draped with the Red Cross flag, it was placed on a gun carriage. Few people saw all this as the public had not been allowed on to the pier, but large crowds watched the procession along the seafront. Many had travelled a very long distance. A Royal Marines band played funeral music and muffled bells rang from the local church. Escorted by the Mayor and councillors, together with twelve women officers and four army nurses, Edith Cavell's body was taken to a waiting railway carriage. Guards kept watch overnight.

The Times of May 16th described the scenes next day as the coffin travelled to London. 'The orchards of Kent were in full blossom, the fields were gold with buttercups, and every bank was blue and white with wild flowers. At almost every station along the line and by the bridges there were crowds of children. They stood in lines three and four deep on the platforms. The boys saluted; the girls stood silently gazing.'

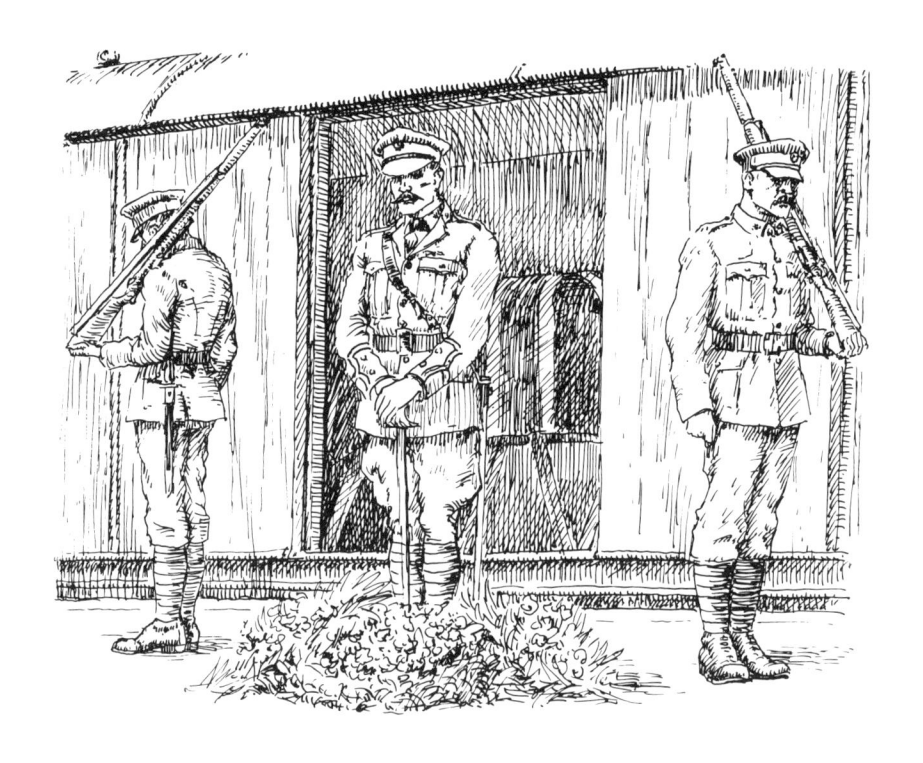

In London, crowds lined the streets all the way from Victoria station to Westminster Abbey, where thousands of people were waiting for the funeral service. They included a representative of King George V and many soldiers. They sang the hymn 'Abide with Me', and Psalm 23 'The Lord is my Shepherd'. Bugles sounded and the coffin, now draped with the Union Jack and topped by a single wreath of red and white flowers, set off for Liverpool Street station. The train left for Norwich at exactly 2.30 p.m.

Two-and-a-half hours later the coffin made the last stage of its journey across the city. It was carried into Norwich Cathedral by eight sturdy sergeant-majors, one of whom had been nursed by Miss Cavell in Belgium. Once again there were masses of flowers. One small bunch had been sent from Bexhill. The card said simply: 'To a noble woman from a humble woman.' Prayers were said, thanking God for Miss Cavell's example of courage and love for other people. The choir sang a beautiful anthem and then the procession moved out of the cathedral through a double line of Red Cross nurses in their blue uniforms. Outside on Life's Green the congregation sang 'Abide with Me' once again, and the coffin was lowered into the ground. *The Times* said: 'No Englishwoman, except Queen Victoria, ever had a more moving or grander progress towards her last resting place.' Today that place is marked by a simple cross and the words: 'To the pure and holy memory of Edith Cavell who gave her life for England. Her name liveth for evermore.'

Edith Cavell had come home.

2 A Norfolk Child

Edith was born only six kilometres from Norwich in the Norfolk village of Swardeston. Although her childhood was a happy one, there was little to suggest that she would one day become a national heroine.

When she was born in 1865, her father, the Rev. Frederick Cavell, had been vicar of Swardeston for two years. Many of his family had been clergymen, and while working in a parish in Islington in North London, he fell in love with Louisa Sophia Warming, the daughter of his housekeeper. They were married in 1863.

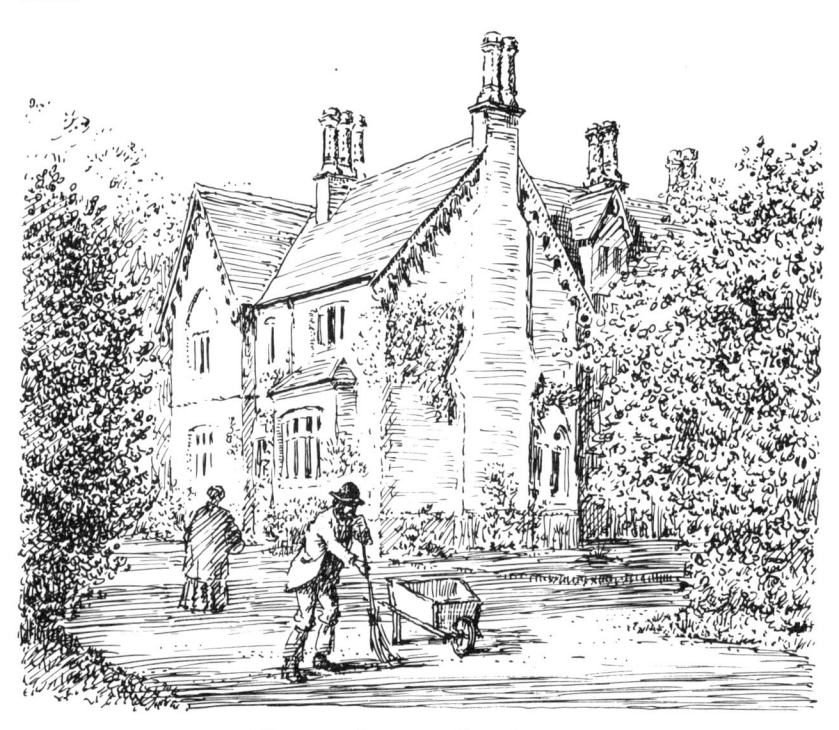

The new vicarage at Swardeston

When they moved to Swardeston, they found that it had no vicarage. But Mr Cavell had recently inherited some money and, being a godly man and keen to help the village, he decided to pay for a new vicarage next to the church. Meanwhile the Cavells lived in a red-brick house on the Common, and it was here that Edith was born. Other children followed — Florence in 1867, Lillian in 1870, and John (known to the family as Jack) in 1873.

The new vicarage was ideal for children. It had large rooms and a lovely garden with a path leading into the churchyard. The Cavells lived comfortably, with a cook, maid and gardener, but they were not able to afford a governess. Men like Frederick Cavell would never have dreamed of sending their children to the village school, so he and his wife taught them at home. Mr Cavell was a strict teacher; the children must have been glad when it was their mother's turn — she was much gentler and the lessons were far more relaxed.

Each day began with family prayers read by Mr Cavell, and on Sundays the children were expected to attend Sunday school, morning and evening services in the church, and evening prayers at home. The children were dressed up in their Sunday best; all toys and non-religious books were locked up until Monday morning. The long hymns and sermons cannot have been very exciting for children. Edith, who was a serious-minded child, never directly rebelled, although she did once write to her cousin Eddy: 'I would love to have you with us, but not on a Sunday. It's too dreadful.'

Mr Cavell was not a man who laughed a great deal,

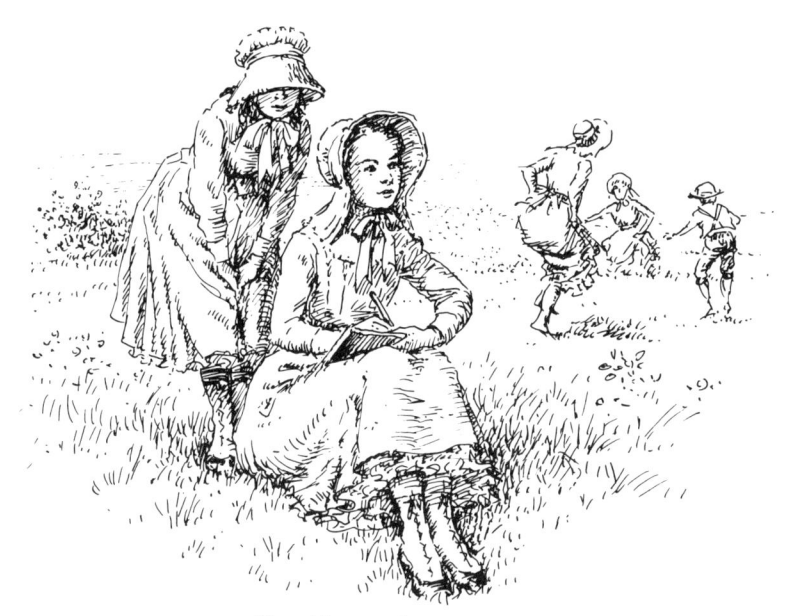

Sketching on the common

although he would sometimes pretend to be a bear and chase after the children. But he was kind and generous to the people of Swardeston. Whenever the family had a hot meal, they shared it. Father carved the joint and the children carried basins of food to the homes of those who were old, ill, or poor. Their own meal must often have been cold by the time they got back.

Life was not all serious. In winter, there was tobogganing and skating on the pond and long walks with the children, dressed from head to foot in flannel to protect them from the wind and rain. In summer, they went blackberry-picking or mushrooming. Edith loved animals, especially dogs, and the family kept lots of pets. She enjoyed sketching, and drew pictures for the younger children and decorated parish notices for her father. She read stories and sang songs to her sisters and brother, and to other children from the village. She also ran errands to the shops, and developed a keen interest in wild flowers; over two hundred varieties grew on the Common. Later the family learned to play tennis and croquet, and Edith collected dolls. There were races, hide and seek, horse-riding and running down the lanes, beating large wooden hoops with a stick.

Each year the Cavells spent their summer holidays at Lowestoft, fifty kilometres away on the Suffolk coast. They shared a rented house with their uncle and aunt from Saxmundham and their three cousins, Frederick, Emmie and Eddy. Eddy was three years older than Edith. Here the children could play on the sands, visit the pier or listen to the band, and take trips by sea along the coast or by train to the Norfolk Broads. Edith and Eddy often went for long walks.

But by 1881 Edith was growing out of the sheltered life of Swardeston and Lowestoft. Her father was furious one day when he found her in his study smoking a cigarette, but he realised that at sixteen she had talents which could not be fully developed at home. They must find the money to send her to school.

Edith had, by now, become a beautiful young lady, short but very slim with soft brown hair and grey eyes full of energy and high spirits. As she prepared to leave home she looked forward to the world which awaited her. She told cousin Eddy: 'Some day I am going to do something useful. It must be something for people. Most of them are so helpless, so hurt, and so unhappy.'

3 A Lovely Girl

Edith did not leave home immediately. In 1881 she attended Norwich High School, probably walking fifteen kilometres each day with her brother Jack who attended another school nearby. After other schools in London and Somerset she went for two years to Laurel Court in Peterborough, run by a fearsome but kindly Irishwoman, Miss Margaret Gibson, in a house near the Cathedral. Miss Gibson loved cats and hated men; only women teachers were employed at Laurel Court.

The school's daily timetable was a strict one — breakfast at 6 a.m., with lessons starting an hour later. During morning break the children ate bread and margarine while walking round the school building in a crocodile. There were no games and discipline was very harsh. Some girls were punished by being shut up in a cupboard; others had to sit cross-legged on the floor with a newspaper over their face. The school encouraged music, especially piano playing. The teachers seem to have been hard-working, but the children were often taught the same lessons over and over again. Edith loved history and literature and had become very interested in French. As well as being a pupil, she was expected to help teach the younger children.

In the summer of 1886 she was in Swardeston, playing tennis and dancing, drawing an album of sketches for her mother and helping to raise money for a Sunday School hall. The vicar had spent all the money he had on the new vicarage, so Edith wrote to the Bishop of

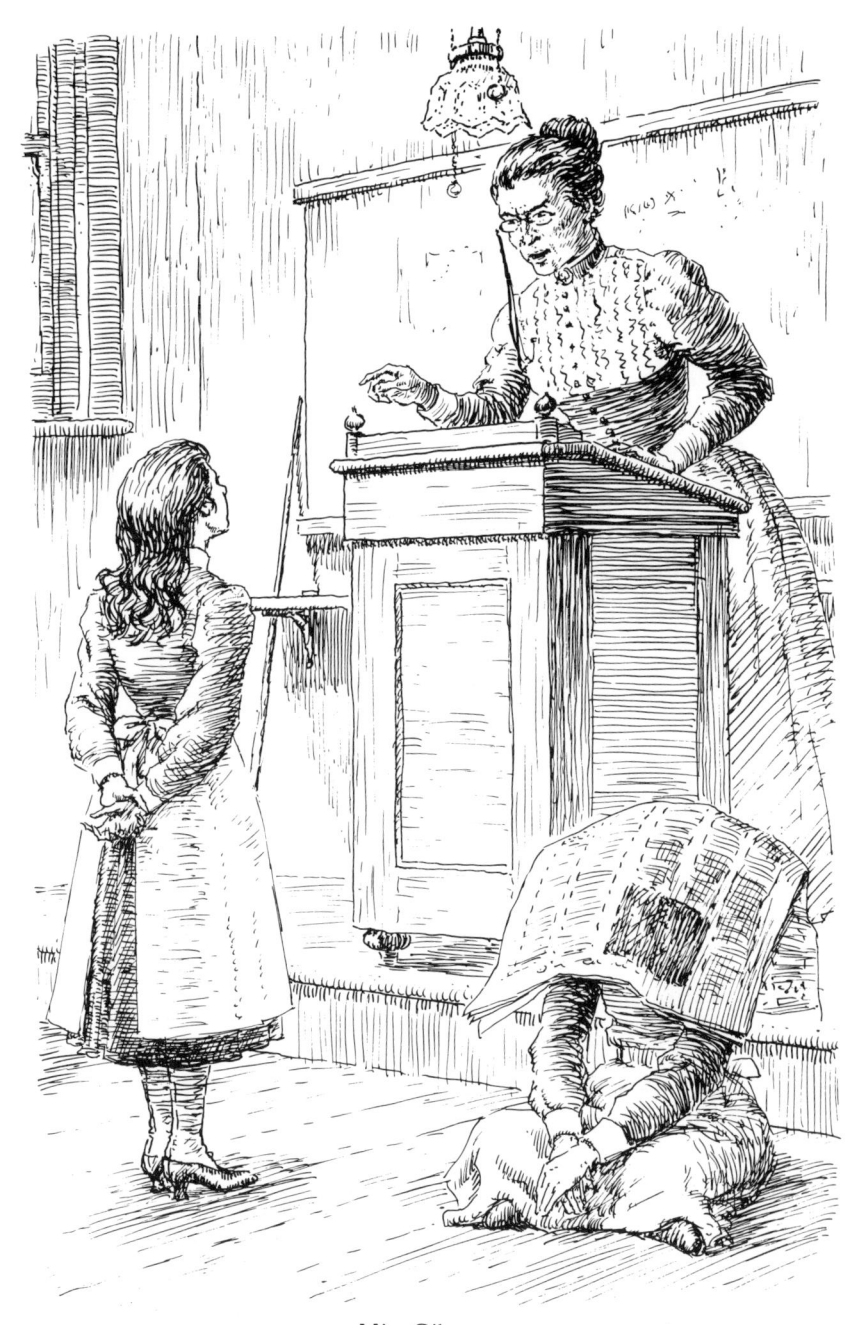

Miss Gibson

Norwich, suggesting that he might help. He replied that if the village could raise part of the money, the Church might be able to provide the rest. Edith promptly organised the family to make Christmas, Easter and birthday cards by the hundreds, which they sold until enough money had been raised to build the hall next to the village stables.

Shortly afterwards she obtained her first job — as governess to the four Powell children. Their father was vicar of an Essex village and their mother was an invalid. Edith gave the children their lessons and organised the food for the household. Each year she took the children to the seaside at Clacton for a month, playing cricket with them on the beach. The whole family came to rely on her and she was adored by the local children. One remembered later: 'She was full of fun and she just loved us. There was always a smile on her face. She was a lovely girl in every way.'

Her time with the Powells ended when the youngest, Jack, went away to school. During 1889-90 she worked in three houses in Norfolk and Essex. When she left one family they gave her a copy of a famous book called *The Imitation of Christ* which, as we shall see, she kept right up to her death.

She was now keen to work abroad, and went to live with the François family in Belgium. M. François was a lawyer who knew Miss Gibson at Laurel Court. Brussels must have been very different from the Norfolk countryside, but Edith stayed there five years. At first she taught the children at home, then later took them to and from school each day. She always spoke English

On the beach at Clacton

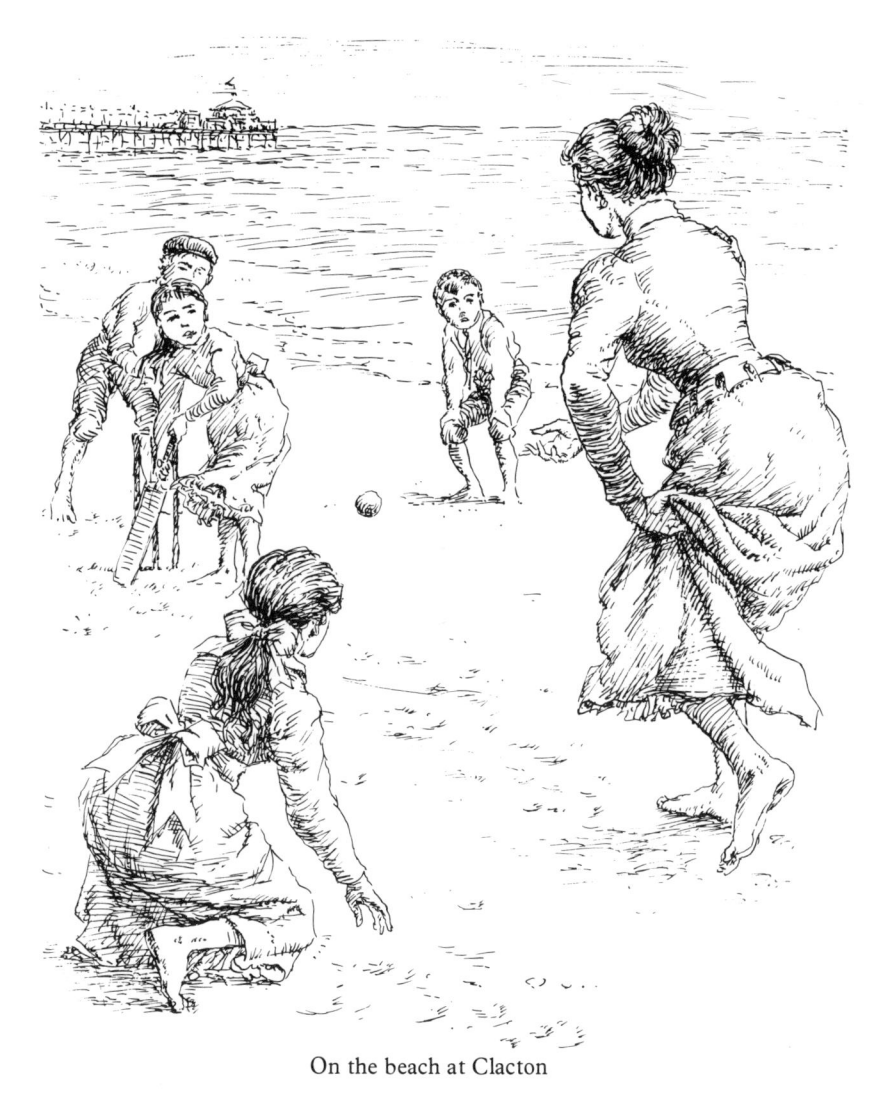

to them, teaching them little plays and nursery rhymes, drawing and painting, how to look after pets and how to collect wild flowers. She also introduced them to English poetry and novels; those of Charles Dickens were her favourites. She could be very strict, especially if the children told lies, and at least once she clashed with their parents. M. François criticised Queen Victoria for having no sense of humour. He may have been joking, but Edith walked out of the room. The children remembered only her kindness, her patience, and the poems she wrote for them. One read —

> Storms may gather, O love, my love,
> But here shall shelter be,
> And in my arms, my dear, my dear,
> The sun shall come back to thee.
>
> The winter of age, O love, my love,
> For us no shade shall bring.
> In thine eyes divine, my dear, my dear,
> For me t'will be always Spring.

Each summer she would go back to Swardeston for a month to see her family again. Helen Swann, a friend of the Cavells, described a tea party at the vicarage in 1892: 'We went into the study after tea to play a very noisy game called 'Animal Grab'. Edith, I remember, was a lion and I was a mouse. I got frightfully excited and made a tremendous noise. In fact, Mr and Mrs Cavell came into the study to see what it was all about. Edith was very amused at my excitement. "Well Helen," she said as we made our departure, "you were very unlike a mouse." '

Edith charmed everyone who met her. Two people in particular fell under her spell. One was Frederick Davey, a difficult boy who had run away from home and who now worked for a local firm. Edith taught him at Sunday School and persuaded him to join the church choir. 'When it was flower time I used to gather a bunch to give to Miss Edith,' he recalled. 'Oh the joy it gave me to make some excuse to go to the Rectory with some little thing, in order just to get one of her smiles and a few kind words.' The other was her cousin, Eddy Cavell. They were always very close, and may even have talked of marriage. But Eddy was a very nervous young man, and perhaps he never dared to propose to her. We cannot be sure. What is certain is that in the thirty years between Edith's death and his own in 1945, he never stopped talking about her.

Edith returned from Brussels in 1895. The François children were growing up now, and her father was seriously ill. Thanks to her care he recovered enough to remain vicar of Swardeston for another fifteen years. But this was a turning point in Edith's life. She was now thirty, and Mr Cavell's illness showed her what she wanted to do. She would become a nurse.

4 The London Hospital

Edith began her nursing career at the Fountains Fever Hospital in Tooting, South London. She worked long hours in a very overcrowded ward. Many of the patients were children and many did not survive. But within three months she was sure that nursing was what she wanted to do, and she was accepted for general training at the London Hospital.

The London Hospital was in the poor East End. Old buildings and a shortage of staff meant that the nurses had to work specially hard. Many of their patients were very old and very poor; some were mentally ill, and others were criminals. It must all have been very

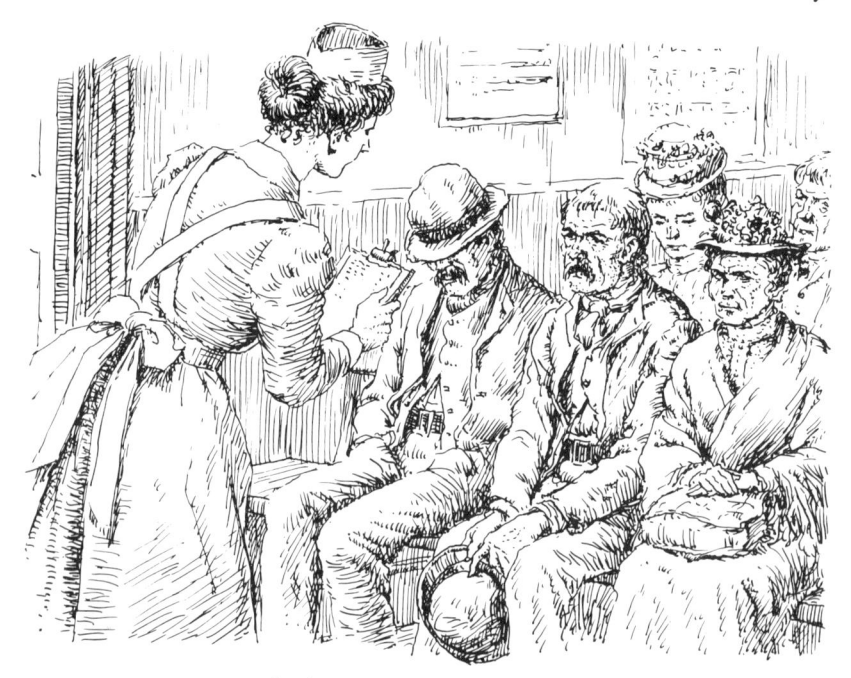

In the outpatients department

different from the comfortable life of a country governess.

However, the doctors were good and the matron, Miss Eva Lückes, was a remarkable woman. She had been there for fifteen years, and had greatly improved the training of the nurses. Edith's interview went well. Miss Lückes liked older girls as trainees, especially if they had done some teaching. A clergyman's daughter was even better. Edith's training began in September 1896.

At first the students did not go near the hospital, but attended lectures and demonstrations instead. Some students changed their minds and left, or were found unsuitable and were told to go. Edith remained, although the report on her was not too encouraging. Some of her tutors found her too sure of herself, and said her work was not thorough enough. She was given a room in the nurses' home, but while she was working during the day her bed was probably slept in by one of the night nurses.

After six weeks she was sent to work on the wards. Breakfast was at 6.30 a.m. each day; she worked from seven in the morning until nine at night with only two hours off, or for eleven hours through the night. She was also expected to attend lectures, and was allowed only two weeks holiday a year. Besides nursing, she was expected to scrub the floors, polish the brasswork and lay the fires in each ward. In her spare time she used to ride around London on the top of a bus or go down the river to Tilbury, but nurses were strictly forbidden to go out with doctors or medical students. If they

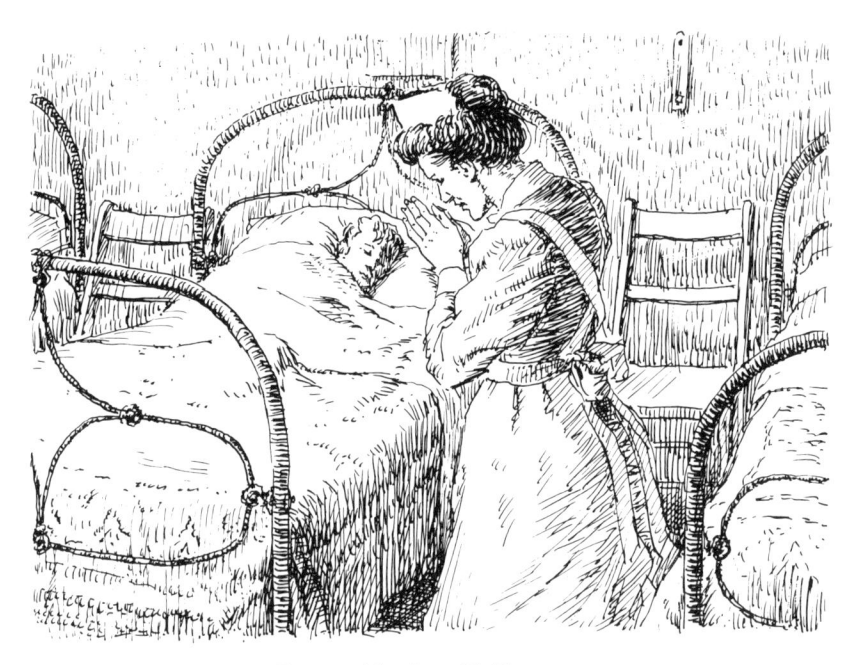

Fever epidemic at Maidstone

disobeyed, the hospital porters would tell Miss Lückes and the nurses would be dismissed at once. A nurse was paid £10 in her first year, rising to £30 two years later.

Hospitals in those days were nothing like they are now. Many of the illnesses which doctors can now deal with, such as diabetes and pneumonia, were incurable. Some diseases, like typhoid and tuberculosis, which were very common then have now almost died out. Anaesthetics (ways of putting a patient to sleep for an operation) were very unpleasant. Far more children died, and far more women lost their lives in childbirth. There were never enough beds for all the patients who needed hospital care. Edith was often seen praying beside the beds of suffering patients.

Miss Lückes expected her nurses to be perfect and she could be very difficult when she thought they had let her down. But she tried to get to know each one individually, and each Tuesday evening she invited any who would like to come to visit her flat for tea and a bun.

In 1897 typhoid fever broke out at Maidstone in Kent, caused by infected water and poor drainage. Emergency hospitals were set up, and nurses were desperately needed. Miss Lückes chose six nurses to go there from the six hundred at the hospital; Edith was one of them. For three months they worked day and night until the fever died down, and were given special medals when they left. A year later Edith passed her hospital certificate. For a time she was sent out of the hospital to nurse patients in their homes, but she was soon brought back to be a staff nurse on one of the wards.

Miss Lückes' reports on Edith during these years are very interesting. They agree that she did good work in Maidstone and say that she was a very capable nurse. But she is criticised for not always being punctual, and for overestimating her own abilities. It is also said that she was not good at working under other people. This was probably true, but it is important also to remember some other facts. Firstly, matrons and sisters in all hospitals were very strict indeed with junior nurses in those days. Secondly, Miss Lückes based her reports on the comments of her ward sisters, some of whom seem to have been rather jealous of Edith, who was older and more self-confident than most of them.

Edith learned a great deal from Miss Lückes and the two wrote to each other for many years. Miss Lückes clearly thought highly of Edith when she sent her to Maidstone, and in 1901 (a few days before Queen Victoria died) she recommended her for the post of night superintendent of the St. Pancras Infirmary, a hospital in another very poor part of London. Edith had a key job here, and she had to take major decisions herself. But the nursing was less interesting than she had been used to, and she missed the bustle of a teaching hospital full of medical students. Besides, she was now thirty-five years old and felt that she wanted a really challenging job, so she began to apply for posts elsewhere.

After several brief jobs her big opportunity came in the summer of 1907. One of Europe's top surgeons, Dr Antoine Depage, asked her to become matron of Belgium's first training school for nurses in Brussels. He wanted an Englishwoman who spoke fluent French and had heard of her through the François family. It was just what Edith was looking for — the chance to build up something entirely new in a country she loved, and to teach others all the nursing skills she had learned herself from Miss Lückes. She accepted at once.

5   The Rue de la Culture

Many people remember Edith Cavell only because of the way she died. But she deserves also to be remembered as the person who, almost alone, began the training of nurses in Belgium.

When she arrived in Brussels in 1907, she found that nursing there was very old-fashioned. In England in the previous fifty years, Florence Nightingale and others had made nursing into a proper profession, quite separate from the training of doctors. Women were proud to be nurses in England; their standard of work was very high, and people respected them greatly. But in Belgium there were no training colleges at all.

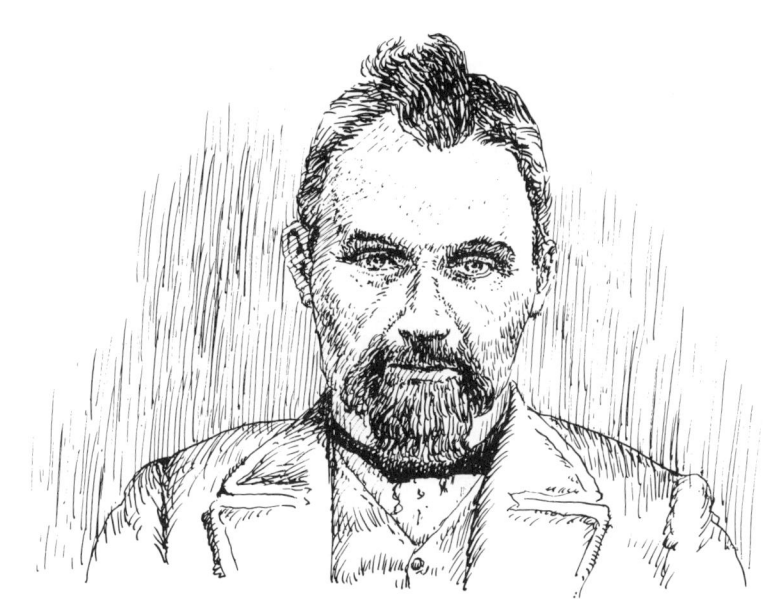

Dr Antoine Depage

Many of the nurses were nuns who knew little about medicine — even those who were expert at caring for the sick might suddenly be withdrawn from a hospital and returned to their convent. And because there were not enough nurses, much of the work in hospitals was done by servants who knew little about the importance of keeping everything clean. Nursing was certainly not a career which Belgians wanted their daughters to take up.

Dr Depage had decided that all this must change. He worked in Brussels University with nurses from abroad and saw that they were much better than the Belgian girls who cared for his patients in the city's hospitals. He was not an easy man to work with, for his temper could sometimes explode without warning. But he and his wife, who got on well with everyone, quickly gained the support of a committee of important people — including the Queen of Belgium. They decided to set up a proper nursing school with its own clinic, and rented four houses in the Rue de la Culture — two for patients' wards and doctors' consulting rooms, and the remainder for the nurses and the matron. There would be about thirty patients at first.

Edith arrived in August. The clinic was due to open on October 1st, but she found that a huge amount still needed to be done. She wrote to Miss Lückes: 'I arrived here two days ago and found the four houses only partly furnished and in much confusion, and the Committee absent on holiday . . . no servants, only a portress.' Four student nurses had been accepted, and only one patient had asked to come so far. 'I never

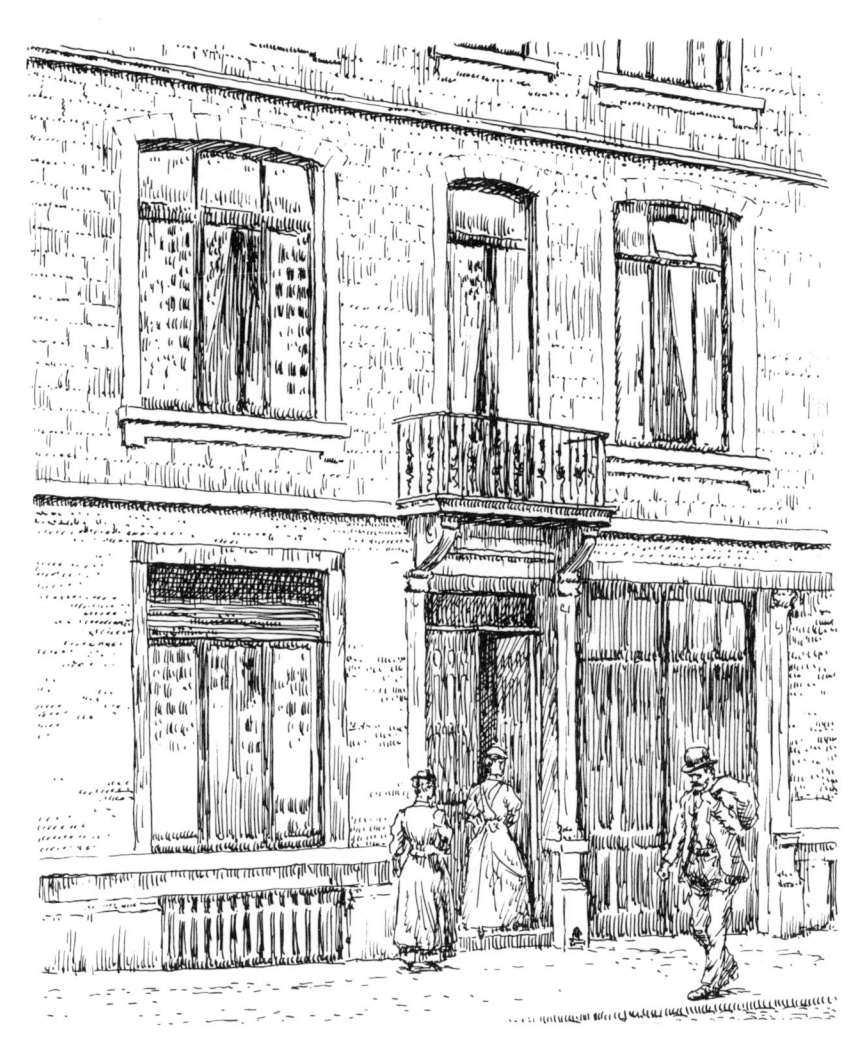

Nursing school in the Rue de la Culture

know from day to day what may happen next and yet I do feel so much depends on these first critical few months,' she remembered later.

Nurses were expected to train in every branch of nursing for three years, and then to work for the school in one of the hospitals with which it had close links. Edith quickly gave the nurses a uniform — blue dresses with white aprons and collars. People nicknamed them 'swallows', because they looked like graceful birds as they hurried from place to place. Her work grew fast, but there were great difficulties. Good nurses were in great demand in Belgium, but poor rates of pay made it difficult to attract really good students and experienced French-speaking nurses from abroad to teach them. Trainee nurses were paid only £7 in their first year and many did not finish the course. Some of the families they worked for treated them very badly. Some of the women Edith interviewed for jobs as servants at the school refused to wait on the nurses, or to serve their meals.

Dr Depage could be very difficult. His language was bad, and Edith once had to refuse him when he asked her to sack a nurse who had been on duty without a proper stiff collar. Nurses thought him rude: 'Do you really expect me to take my hat off and bow every time I see you?' he asked one who had complained to Edith. 'No, but you can at least say good morning,' she replied. He quickly learned, and often presented them with chocolates and gingerbread. The Committee knew little about nursing. When the first students refused to do night duty for more than a week at a time instead of the month that Edith wanted, Committee members forced her to agree — although the nurses themselves later came to see that Edith was right. 'They are on the whole very nice,' wrote Edith to Miss Lückes about the Committee, 'but a few are anxious to limit my authority.

Some even object to my offering tea to people who call!' And there was a continual shortage of money for improvements. There were no lifts; water for sterilising had to be boiled in saucepans, and patients ready for operations had to be carried out of one house and into the one next door by way of the street. Some patients took a very long time to pay their bills.

But Edith never lost her temper. She built the clinic into a nursing centre of major importance. There were sixty nurses by 1912, working in nearly fifty hospitals and other centres in the city. By the time that the first nurses completed their three-year training in 1910, the Belgian government had introduced a scheme to make a national register of all nurses who had been properly trained — a sign of how important they thought Edith's work was. Edith gave her own nurses a special badge when they finished their training.

In 1912 the Committee began to raise funds to build a new, modern clinic and school in the centre of Brussels. 'The Belgian school of nursing has been an entire success,' commented Dr Depage. By the summer of 1914 the building was quickly taking shape. Unfortunately, Edith did not live to see it finished.

6 A Loyal Friend

What was life like at Edith's clinic? She wrote a description for the *Nursing Mirror* in 1908 saying; 'The nurses will build a career here which demands the best and highest qualities that womanhood can offer.' But the work came as a great shock to many of the girls. They worked nine hours a day, six and a half days a week. After a two-month trial period they were expected to sign on for five years. The trial period was deliberately very tough. One nurse recalled: 'I had been brought up in a home where all work of that kind was done by domestic servants. I had never seen my mother or elder sisters cleaning anything, except possibly the best silver. In January I joined the school, and was immediately told to help nurse in one of the small wards. There I had to watch the patients, clean and dust, and carry meals on trays up three flights of stairs. I remember having to mop the floors. Matron came round every day soon after ten o'clock. She would often put a finger on the top of a wardrobe, or on a bar under a bed and, if she found a speck of dust, would say quietly but reprovingly "Dusting must be finished by ten o'clock, nurse." '

Perhaps it is therefore not surprising that the nurses lived in great awe of Edith. 'Miss Cavell required obedience to her orders, and I never met a nurse who dared to disobey her,' said one. 'Her remarks were often severe, and we never dared to be late for meals, knowing that we would encounter the stern reproach of her grey eyes and the hard expression of her lips. We would often be called to her office to be told off for laughing too loudly, or to be warned to be more careful about our manners.'

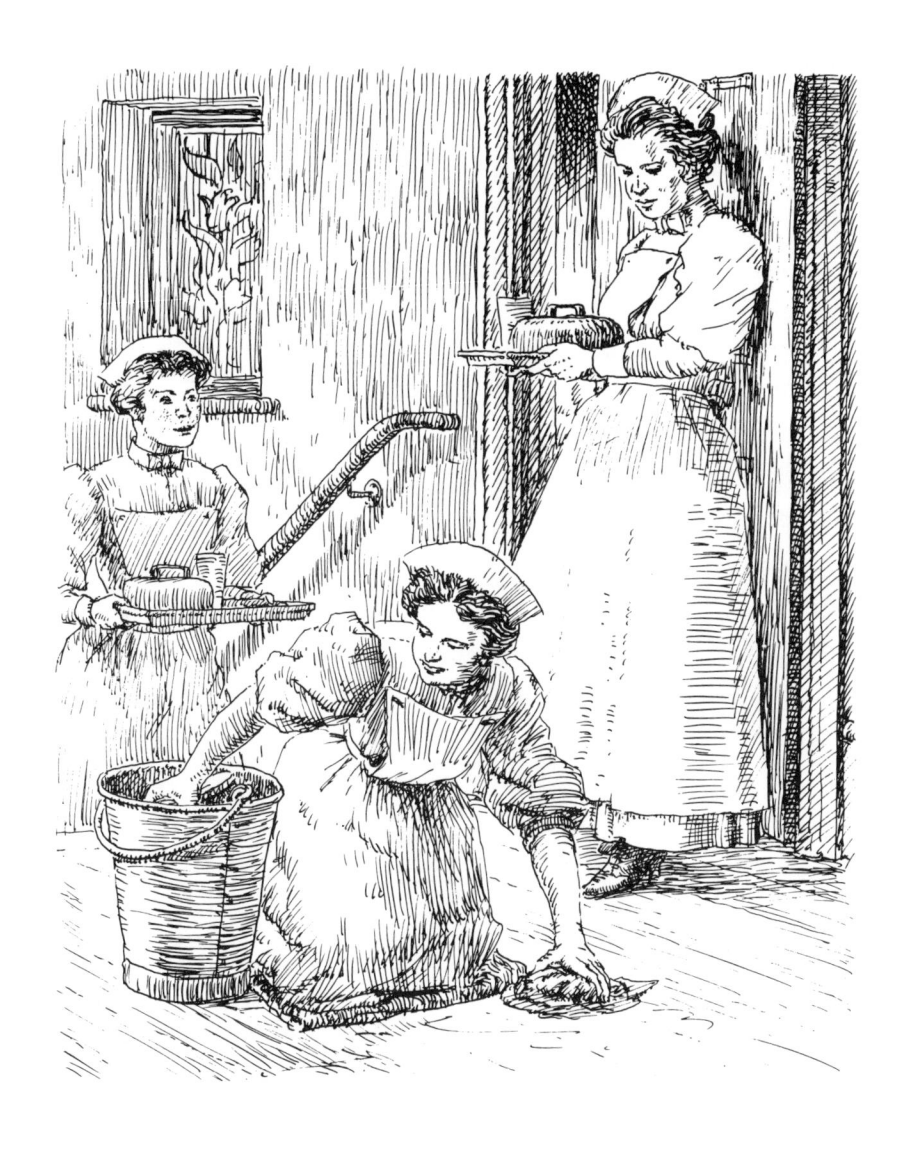

The discipline was certainly very strict. If the nurse was more than two minutes late for breakfast, she lost her two free hours during the day — even though Edith had often been unpunctual as a young nurse herself. Nurses were not allowed to receive presents from patients, and could not talk to a doctor except about a patient. Once a nurse had taken a patient on, she could never give him up, however badly she was treated.

Some girls found all this rather too much. They could not understand Edith's enormous sense of duty, and she seemed a lonely figure to them with few, if any, friends. She had few relaxations — even occasional visits to the theatre had stopped by 1914. She would sometimes play hymns on the piano after evening lectures, but she seemed very distant, even from her senior staff. Her religion was certainly very strong. 'Never in the whole seven years that I knew Miss Cavell did I ever hear her laugh,' wrote one doctor. Another recalled that 'she seemed a very quiet character and spoke very little. She seldom smiled.' At times she seemed to take life too seriously for some people. 'A woman does not take life, she gives it,' she told a student who was about to crush a spider with her foot.

But Edith expected from her nurses only the high standards she kept to herself. She worked amazingly hard. Breakfast at 7.00 a.m. with her students, her watch out on the table, followed by a meeting with her senior nurses to plan the day. She attended every operation and every lecture given by the doctors. After lunch she would often lecture herself, and did so very well indeed. She went round all the hospitals which she supplied with nurses every day. She joined the nurses for dinner

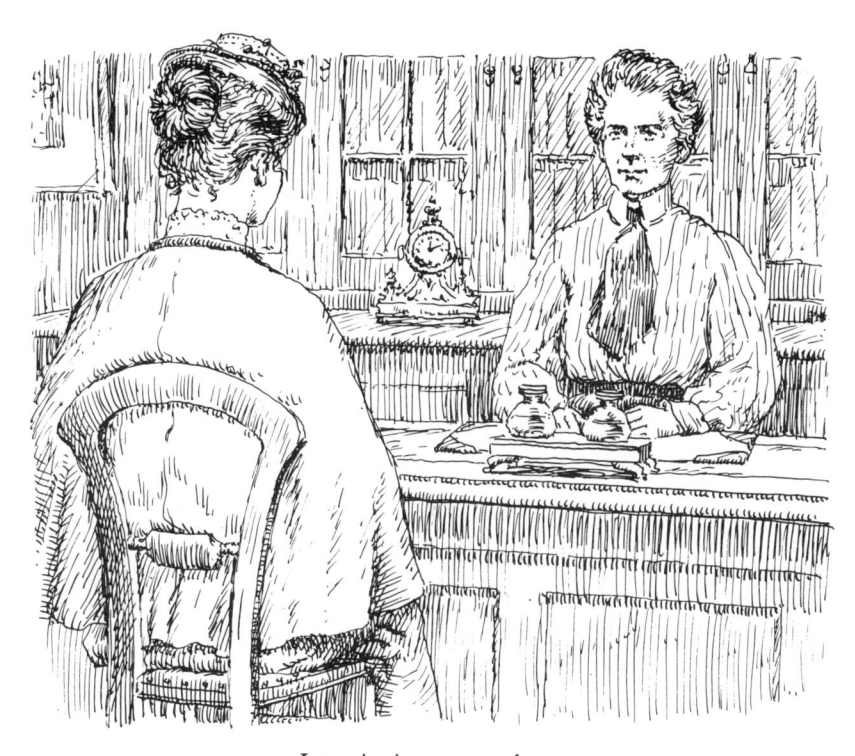

Interviewing new students

at 7 each night, having usually seen a series of callers in her room. At the end of the meal, the nurses bowed to her silently and left without speaking. In the evening reports were brought to her office and difficult cases were discussed. After that, she might well talk to a group of nurses before bed. And some time during the day she had to interview possible new students, prepare a lecture, or write a newspaper article.

Edith kept two dogs — Don, the mongrel died in 1912 but Jack, a collie, was still alive when she died. She kept them spotlessly clean and walked them regularly, much to the annoyance of the students whom she often found up to mischief. 'Miss Cavell had her spies everywhere,' said one. Two of the people they thought of as spies were Grace Jemmett and Pauline Randall. Grace Jemmett, addicted to the drug morphine as a result of a serious illness, was sent to the clinic by Dr Wainwright, Edith's brother-in-law, who hoped her strong discipline might bring about a cure. Grace became like a daughter to Edith, and even called her 'Mother'. The money which her wealthy family paid for her to be a patient was very welcome but nothing could cure her; she became increasingly helpless and would do anything to get more drugs. This embarrassed Edith and annoyed the nurses. Pauline Randall had run away from a circus at the age of thirteen, and was sent to Edith by the English chaplain in Brussels. 'We did not take kindly to Pauline. She would report us to her mistress for the slightest error in our duties,' said one nurse.

Certainly at times Edith seems to have expected too much. Even in 1913 with so many achievements to her credit, she wrote to Miss Lückes: 'The young girls are brought up with no sense of duty. They are selfish and too fond of pleasure.' On the other hand she could be very kind and understanding. One nurse was sent to stay with Edith's sister in Henley to recover from a persistent illness. A Dutch student caught dancing in a night club when off duty was allowed to remain, and later went on to supervise another hospital. Edith loved sharing her experience with visitors from other countries, and the children's ward was always the highlight of her hospital rounds. Eileen Humfrey was brought into the clinic with scarlet fever at the age of nine. 'She made me a nurse's uniform, and I was terribly proud of it,' Eileen remembered. Edith also persuaded the doctors to pretend they thought Eileen was a real nurse.

She did have a sense of humour. The nurses were often invited to tea with Mme Depage, the doctor's wife, but there was very little food. They always came back hungry. When they asked Edith for more, she pretended to be surprised but then said: 'All right, I think you had better all have tea with me,' and gave them a large wink. Once a student forgot to turn off a bath and water came pouring down the stairs. The nurses rushed to clear it up before Edith arrived and tried to keep her away from the area. 'She turned back,' remembered one, 'but with that twinkle in her eyes. I am sure she had taken in the situation and liked us for our spirit.' Two days later when she met the students in the linen room below the bathroom, everything still smelled horribly of damp. Edith looked at the ceiling, then at the nurses and said — nothing.

The nurses greatly admired her. Some of them even came to love her dearly. One staff nurse noted that she was 'cold in her manner, but a staunch and loyal friend in times of trouble.' By the summer of 1914, Edith was forty-eight but looked a lot older. Perhaps her sense of duty was driving her too hard. That summer she went

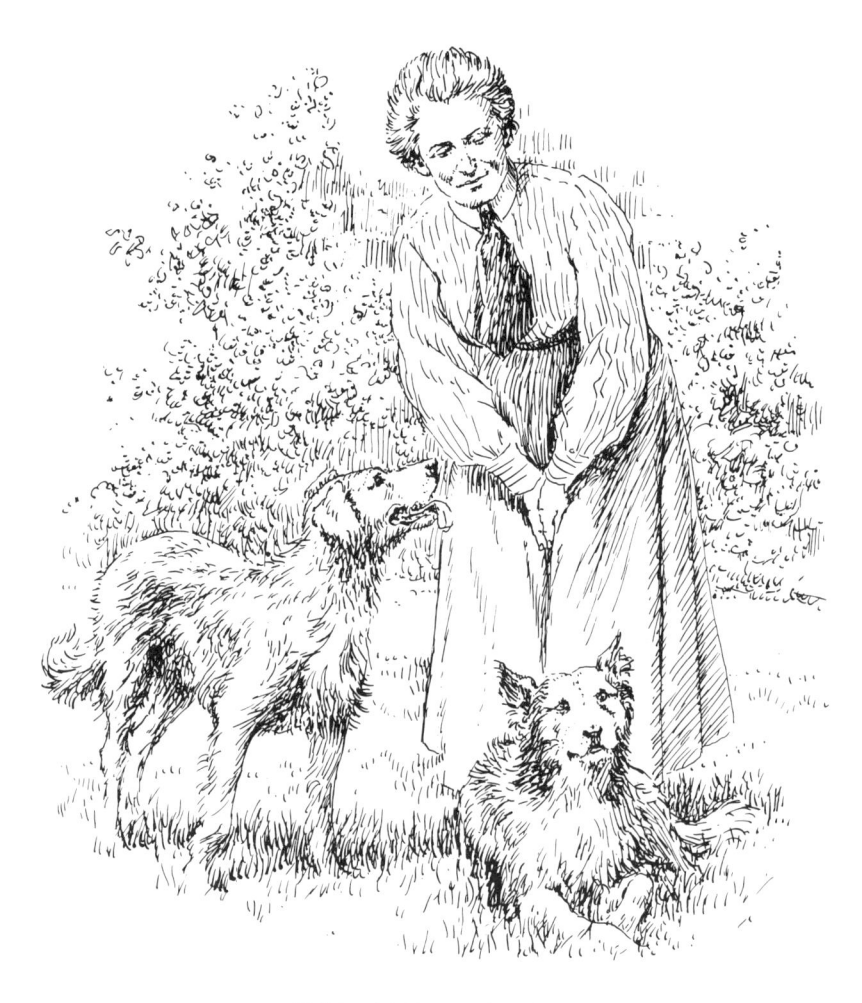

Edith with Don and Jack

home to Norfolk for her usual holiday. Her mother had been living in Norwich since Mr Cavell's death four years earlier, and Edith always tried to be there on Mrs Cavell's birthday — July 6th. A little later she went to stay with old friends on the coast at West Runton. It was a beautiful hot summer. While in Norfolk, there was very serious news from across the Channel.

7 War

On June 28th 1914 the heir to the Austrian throne, Archduke Francis Ferdinand, was shot dead in the city of Sarajevo. The murderer had come across the border from Serbia (now Yugoslavia); a month later the Austrians declared war. The Russians quickly prepared to protect Serbia. Germany was Austria's ally and France had treaties with Russia; by early August war was a certainty.

Germany had always been afraid of wars at the same time against Russia to the East and France to the West. Knowing that Russia would take a long time to come to battle, the Germans decided to knock France out first. But the quickest way into France lay across the flat land of Belgium. The Germans marched into Belgium on August 2nd and the British, who had promised to protect Belgium, joined the war.

Edith quickly left Norfolk. In a few days a friend recorded: 'Miss Cavell was back at the clinic quite ready for the wounded, and Red Cross flags hung all over the house.' Her German nurses had to go home, although her German maid Marie was allowed to stay — we do not know why.

Edith wrote several newspaper articles describing events in Belgium. At first, everyone was cheerful in Brussels; flags flew everywhere in the streets; people welcomed the war, and were sure that the British and French would save them. Edith was desperately busy, caring for all the wounded in a hospital which was now very short of staff. But after the Germans destroyed the

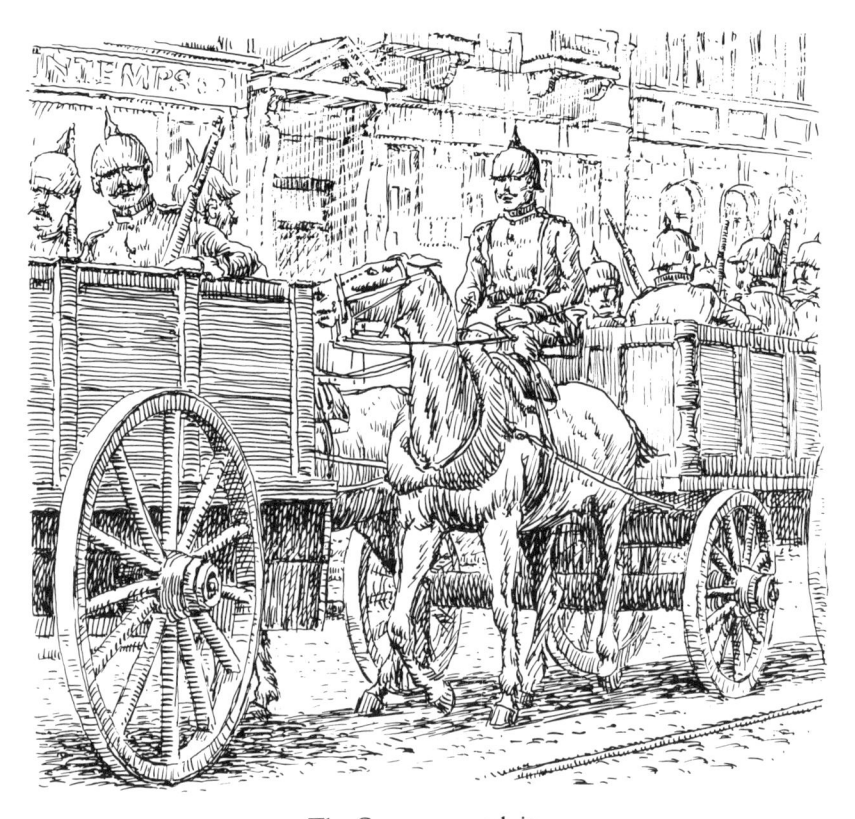

The Germans march in

city of Louvain, the Belgian king ordered that Brussels was not to resist. All the sick and wounded fled, and many of the hospitals were closed. Edith wrote to her mother on August 19th: 'The Germans are very close here. We expect the worst.' That evening she called her nurses together and told them that it was their duty to nurse all the wounded, friend or enemy.

The Germans entered Brussels next day. Edith wrote: 'The troops were all in grey . . . some were too weary to eat and slept on the pavement. We were divided between pity for these poor fellows, far from their country and people, suffering the weariness of an arduous campaign, and hate of a cruel foe bringing ruin to a peaceful land.' But once the fighting moved away from Brussels, life became much quieter. Newspapers were censored, trains and telephones were to be used only by Germans, and nobody was allowed on the streets at night. Spies were everywhere. Nevertheless, the people were treated quite well on the whole. The fighting was now fifty kilometres to the south-west. On August 23rd the British fought a desperate battle at Mons as they tried to delay the German advance.

Edith probably wrote a hundred letters home during the war. They had to be sent secretly and many of them never got through. We now have eighteen of them, mostly to her mother. In late August she was writing: 'I cannot give you details of things here. We are in the dark. The wildest rumours are current — we know for certain that there is fighting near at hand because we can hear the cannon. We have a few German wounded in our hospital but the allies are not brought to Brussels. There has been terrible loss of life on both sides.' A month later: 'Everything is quiet at our end of the town. There is plenty of food at the moment. We are busy making clothes for the poor; there will be great need of them this winter — there are so many refugees and so many homeless. There is very little coal.'

This must have been a very frustrating time. Edith had refused to go home because she thought that there would be so much work to do in Belgium. But now there seemed to be none. Suddenly, on November 1st, everything changed.

8   A Higher Duty than Prudence

Late on November 1st 1914 Sister Millicent White, one of Edith's nurses, was standing in the room across the corridor from Edith's office. She was reading a copy of *The Times*. Although it was over two weeks old and therefore very out of date, it was very precious. People in Brussels were not supposed to read about the fighting — especially from a newspaper produced in England. Copies were very hard to get; the paper normally sold for one penny but Edith had paid £5 for it.

Sister White quickly hid the paper when she heard a knock at the door. Marie let in three men. Sister White thought perhaps they were German policemen, until she noticed that two of them were very poorly dressed. Marie went into Edith's office and soon came back to take the three men in to see her. A few minutes later the well-dressed man, Herman Capiau, left very hurriedly.

Shortly afterwards Edith came to find Sister White. 'This is Colonel Boger and Sergeant Meakin,' she said. 'They have both been wounded. You will look after them, won't you, and give them a meal? And you will see that they have some beer?' Sister White took them to the house next door, gave them food, and bandaged up their wounds.

The two men were members of the 1st Cheshire Regiment. Heavily outnumbered at Mons, the British army had quickly retreated westwards. Many soldiers and regiments lost touch with each other, and rapidly found themselves trapped in areas full of German

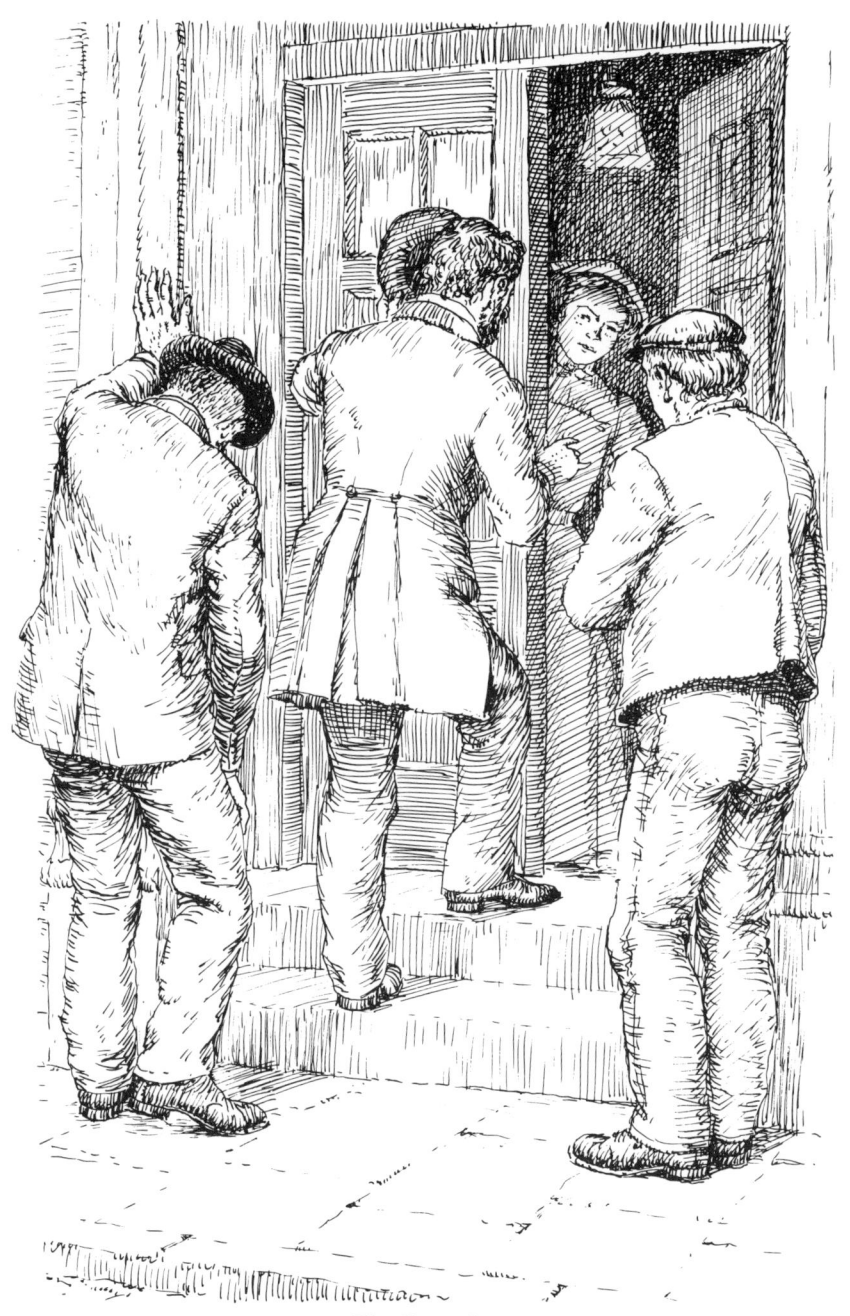

The first refugees

soldiers. Colonel Boger had injuries to his hand, his side, and his right foot. Sergeant Meakin had been hit on the head by a spent bullet, and by a piece of shrapnel rebounding off a tree. Both had been captured, and taken to a field hospital; but they had managed to escape, and were given shelter by Albert Libiez, a Mons lawyer, who became a leading figure in the Resistance movement. Boger had now grown a beard, and was wearing a black hat and floppy tie like many Belgians of the time, while Meakin had disguised himself as a labourer, and was wearing shoulder pads to make him look like a hunchback.

Both men hoped to escape to England by way of Brussels and Holland; however, the Germans had declared that any British soldiers who did not surrender, and anyone who helped them, would be shot. Boger's foot injury was very bad, and it seemed likely that he might die unless he got urgent medical help. He and Meakin were brought to Brussels and it was Mme Depage who had suggested that Edith might help.

Boger and Meakin stayed at the clinic for two weeks. Gradually Edith began to fear that the house was being watched, so she arranged for them to be taken to another house in the city from where Boger, who was still very lame, was to travel to the Dutch coast on a coal barge, while Meakin would travel by land to meet him. Although deserted by his guide, Meakin managed to get to England, but Boger was captured and became a prisoner for most of the war. Sister White, who went home via Antwerp shortly afterwards on a false

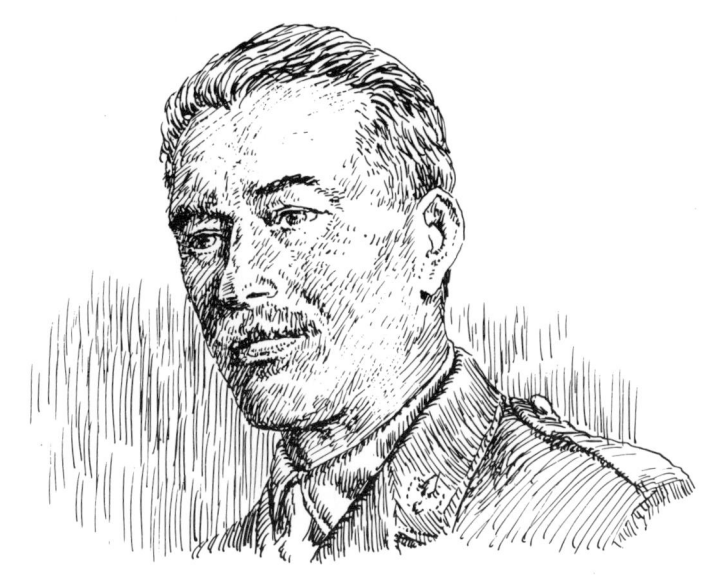

Colonel Boger

passport, took important papers from the Colonel bandaged around her leg.

Edith's letters home show little of all this excitement. She did, however, admit 'We have had some interesting work but are quiet again now. Our people who left last week must have arrived safely as they have not returned.' Maybe she thought such hints would help her family to guess what was happening. Otherwise the letters talk of how poor and hungry many people were, of preparing for Christmas, and of how much she looked forward to her next holiday in Norfolk.

Edith seems to have had only a moment to decide whether to take in the two soldiers or to send them away, probably to their deaths. She took a brave decision but a very dangerous one. As she said: 'In times like these, there is a higher duty than prudence.' There could be no going back now.

9 I Cannot Express Enough Thanks

Edith and the clinic became part of an organised Resistance movement. We shall never know exactly how many men passed through her hands, but the total may be four hundred or even many more. Some stayed several weeks, others only a day or two. Many people risked their lives in helping the operation — like the clinic's Rumanian porter José, who often carried the wounded up and down stairs. Others included an architect, Philippe Baucq, who helped to distribute a secret newspaper, and who drew sketches of airship bases for English agents to take home. Prince Reginald de Croy and his sister Princess Marie owned the castle of Bellignies, not far from Mons. They hid many soldiers in secret rooms, and Marie took photographs for their false passports. Some of these were developed by a local chemist and Resistance worker, Louis Severin. A schoolteacher, Louise Thuliez, brought many of the men to the clinic, and helped them with the next stage of their journey from there. Many others hid escapers in their houses. Most, like Edith, were keen Christians.

The soldiers had remarkable tales to tell, although some kept quiet until after Edith's death in case news should get back to the Germans. Sergeant Tunmore — who knew Norfolk well — and Private Lewis had their passport photos taken by Edith herself. She personally took them on the first stage of their escape. Sergeant Tunmore later wrote to Mrs Cavell: 'I cannot express enough thanks for all that she has done for me.'

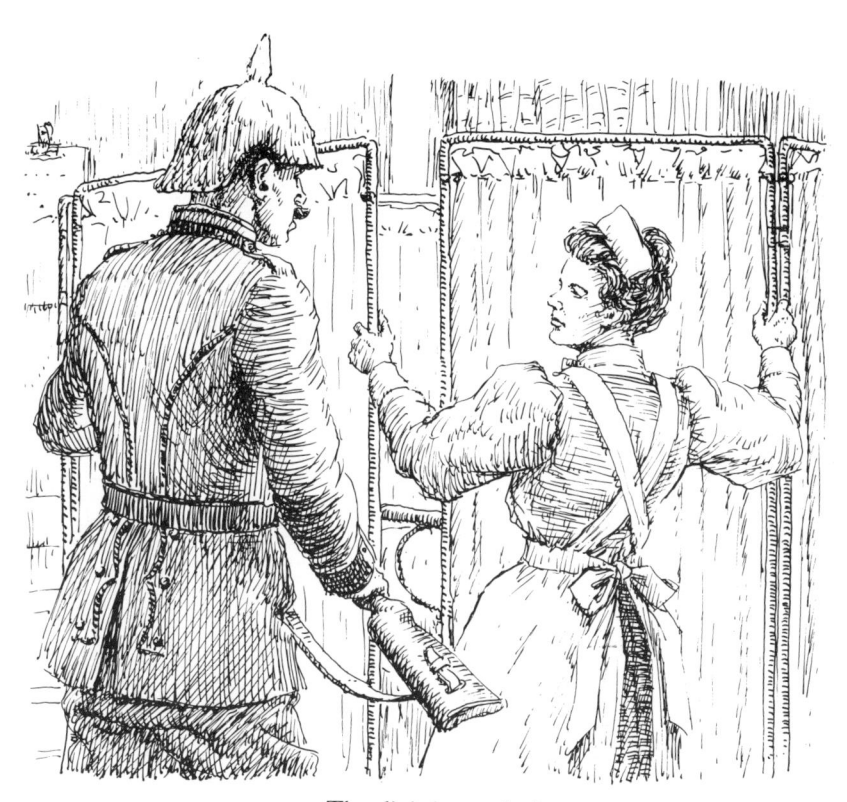

The clinic is searched

Lance-corporal Doman and Corporal Chapman stayed two weeks. The Germans visited the clinic unexpectedly while they were there, and Doman was quickly pushed into a bed, still wearing his army boots. Later Edith contacted a guide, and took them to a café to find him. She had never met him, but laid half a visiting card down on the table. The guide soon came in with the other half.

Private Wood worked as a ward orderly during his time at the clinic. When the Germans arrived, he undressed and got into bed; screens were put round the bed, and they took no notice. Lance-Corporal Holmes

47

lived in Norwich, only a few minutes' walk from Mrs Cavell's house. He carried Edith's Bible back to England with a letter for her mother; he delivered both, but unfortunately Mrs Cavell panicked, and refused to see him when he called.

Privates Heath and Beaumont were housed in an attic, with nearly twenty other soldiers. Beaumont later escaped with Private Grey, who had gone out for an evening from his previous hiding-place and returned only to find the owner and eleven other soldiers executed and the house burned down. Private Scott arrived at the clinic very ill. One night Edith woke him up and said 'I am in trouble. You will have to come with me.' He was hidden in a barrel of apples until the Germans had finished their search.

Edith was amazingly brave and cheerful. One man arrived at the clinic and was given a form to sign for an operation. 'There must be some mistake,' he said, 'I thought you were going to help me cross the frontier.' 'That, Monsieur, is the operation,' said Edith with a broad smile. Private Robert Mapes came from Hethersett, almost the next door village to Swardeston. 'Dear old Norfolk,' she exclaimed when she found out, 'I would do anything to help a Norfolkman.' Then she kissed him. Corporal Sheldrake, to whom Edith gave a shirt for his escape, thought her so wonderful that he asked to be buried in it when he died.

The risks were increasing all the time. Men were coming to the clinic in very large numbers. The Germans set up a command post in a house opposite. Edith knew that there must be informers amongst the guides, but some of the soldiers didn't understand that there were spies everywhere. They got very bored while hidden away, so she let them go out in small groups in the evenings. One night a group of them got drunk, and came back down the street singing 'It's a long way to Tipperary' very loudly. The next day at dawn they were all sent away to other houses in case the Germans had heard.

Edith must have known that it was only a matter of time before she would be arrested. She kept a photograph album of many of the soldiers she had helped. She also kept a diary. Some sheets of it were hidden in a cushion and were only discovered thirty years later. They are now in the Imperial War Museum in London.

Perhaps sensing that the end was near, her letters began to contain bigger hints. In March 1915 she wrote to cousin Eddy: 'There are many things that I may not write until we are again free. Do you think you could find out news of the soldiers on the enclosed list? They are relations of some of the girls here.' The list included names of men she had helped to escape. She ended: 'I like to look back on the days when we were young and life was fresh and beautiful.'

The final letters to her mother include warnings to prepare for the worst. 'People are often arrested without warning . . . Marie has been giving me a good deal of trouble . . . Do not forget that if anything very serious should happen you could probably send a message through the American ambassador in London . . .' Some weeks later, the blow was to fall.

10 Arrest

By July 1915 the situation at the clinic had become very tense indeed. It was now being watched all the time. On June 20th two men called on Edith, saying they would like to rent the houses when the clinic moved to its new buildings. They insisted on being shown all round and took great interest in the water tanks in the bathroom. Around the same time there had been a serious police raid while Edith was out. 'Have you any more?' was all the visitor would say when Sister Wilkins asked him what he wanted — and then he showed her his badge with the words 'Secret Political Police'. She delayed him long enough for José to hide two soldiers who were in one of the wards. When he asked to see Edith's office, papers which might have proved her guilt had already been quickly stuffed into the cistern of the lavatory on the landing. Edith burned many of them when she got back.

She became especially suspicious of George Gaston Quien, a Frenchman. He was a great nuisance at the clinic and she finally got him away on June 30th. He soon came back, saying that he wanted to work for French Intelligence instead of escaping, but she refused to let him in again.

On July 31st Louise Thuliez and Philippe Baucq were arrested at Baucq's house. Quien had been seen outside a little earlier. Five days later a plain-clothes police inspector came to stay in the room opposite Edith's office. On the following afternoon, police ransacked the office and took Edith away. Princess

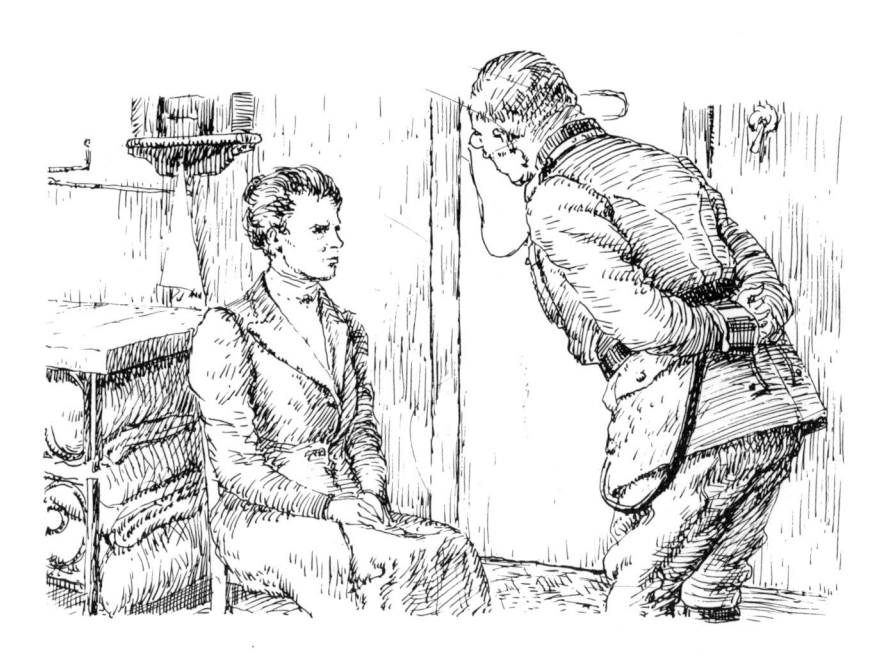

Marie was arrested on September 6th.

After two days at police headquarters Edith was taken to St Gilles prison. She was well-treated; the food was reasonable and she was allowed to send letters out, but the corridors were patrolled day and night and the cell was small. She made two beautiful table mats, and read her little *Imitation of Christ* over and over again, underlining such sentences as 'Be thou prepared for the fight if thou wilt have victory.' She wrote several letters to her nurses: 'I am happy to know that you are working well for some of you must shortly sit for your examinations. Au revoir, be really good.' Meanwhile, Sister Wilkins was organising the move to the clinic's new buildings which were at last complete.

Edith was questioned at great length by the Germans. Some people have suggested that she gave away full details of the escapes and of those involved, believing that one must always tell the truth. But Sister Wilkins said later that Edith had always said that if either of them were questioned, they were to say nothing. It now seems much more likely that she told the Germans only facts that she was sure they knew already from informers like Quien.

The Germans wanted the world to believe that she had deliberately betrayed her friends. Some also believed that they tricked her into overestimating the amount they knew, and that they made up many of the 'facts' she is supposed to have given them. She spoke in French, while police took notes in German and read them back to her in French. But she had to sign the German version without being able to understand the paper she was actually signing. The notes may even have been rewritten later, and Edith's signature forged on them. She is supposed to have said that only two or three of the soldiers she sheltered were wounded, but we know that many of them were severely injured. To deny that would only have made her case worse. The Germans also claimed that she was the only one of those arrested to sign a statement. This was probably said to excuse her death; it is certainly not true. To have deliberately betrayed her friends would have been quite unlike her.

On October 3rd 1915 seventeen nurses from the clinic sent a letter to the German Governor-general in Belgium saying that Edith had done outstanding work at the clinic, and begging for her release. But the Germans had already fixed the date of her trial. It was to begin only four days later.

11 They Want My Life

The trial opened on October 7th. The Germans had chosen their aggressive prosecution lawyer, Dr Stoeber, very carefully; defence lawyers, who had to be approved by the Germans, had not been allowed to see or write to the accused beforehand and did not know the precise charges they would face. German hatred of England was very strong now, because the war was not going well for Germany. A new Military Governor of Brussels had just been appointed. He was known to be very severe.

The prisoners were brought from the gaol in an ancient van, packed like sardines. There were thirty-five of them. Some had been guides, or had organised escapes; some were chemists who had developed passport photographs, and others had provided shelter for the escapers. The most important prisoners were placed directly in front of the judges, guarded by German soldiers with bayonets fixed. There were five judges — all in military uniform — and the court was filled with German officers. Almost no Belgian spectators were allowed in.

When the charges had been read, the other prisoners were taken out and Edith was questioned. She was asked only twelve questions, and gave very little away. She said that her only aim had been to help those men who came to her to reach the frontier. Questioning of the other prisoners followed. They were quietly defiant. Princess Marie declared: 'One must do one's duty without thinking of the consequences,' and claimed that she had been forced to say some of the things that were included in her statement to the police. She also believed that some of the prisoners had been drugged to make them tell more of what they knew.

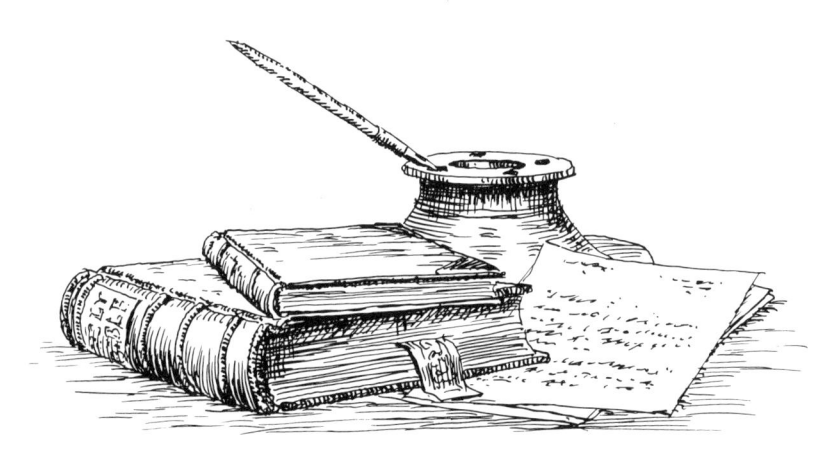

At noon the judges disappeared and huge saucepans of soup and coffee were brought in for the guards. No food was provided for the prisoners, although a few guards offered them some. Edith whispered to Louise Thuliez that she thought things looked very bad for them — 'but what does it matter so long as we are not shot?'

In the afternoon the prosecution called its two witnesses. One declared that all the prisoners had been questioned fairly, and said they all belonged to one organisation determined to harm the German war effort. The surprise witness was the fourteen-year-old son of one of the accused. He was threatened with ten years hard labour unless he told the truth, and he gave evidence especially damaging against Philippe Baucq.

Next day Stoeber spoke for three and a half hours. He demanded the death sentence for nine of the prisoners. Soon the trial was over; sentences would be announced to the accused in prison later. Three days of waiting followed. Edith read the Bible and her *Imitation of Christ*. On one chapter, about the need to call on God for help in difficult times, she wrote 'St Gilles 1915'. On Monday afternoon the prisoners were called together, and told that five of them were to die. Edith was one of them. One of the prisoners urged her: 'Madame, make an appeal for mercy.' 'It is useless,' she replied calmly. 'I am English and they want my life.' They were taken back to the cells.

The Germans tried to keep the sentences secret, fearing a wave of unpopularity. But rumours soon leaked out. Nurses went to the prison, but were not allowed in. The Germans told Belgian lawyers that the judgements had not yet been announced. But one member of the American embassy went with the Spanish ambassador to see the German political minister, Baron von der Lancken. He was at the theatre, and refused to leave until the play had finished, but he seemed amazed at Edith's sentence, and at rumours that she was to be shot at dawn next day. Eventually he agreed to contact the Military Governor, but it was no good. Von der Lancken probably realised that killing Edith would do Germany's reputation abroad great harm, but one of the other officers merely said that he wished they had several other old English women to shoot as well.

The Military Governor had decided that two of the accused, Edith Cavell and Philippe Baucq, should indeed die at once. The Belgian prison chaplain broke the news to Edith that Monday afternoon.

12 Brussels: Dawn; October 12th

Edith remained completely controlled when she heard the news. The priest asked if she would like the British chaplain in Brussels to be with her at her execution. 'Oh no,' she replied, 'Mr Gahan isn't used to things like that.' But she did agree to see him that evening. She was not allowed any other visitors.

Mr Gahan, dreadfully shocked at the sentence, arrived at the jail at 8.30 in the evening. 'She is a fine character,' the German warder told him. He went in to see her. 'All anxieties were set to rest in a moment,' he recalled. 'There she stood, her bright, gentle, cheerful self, as always, quietly smiling, calm and collected, even cheerful. She gave me a kind and grateful welcome.'

They took Communion, prayed and said the hymn 'Abide with Me'. They talked a little. 'I have no fear,' she said, 'I have seen death so often that it is not strange to me. Life has always been hurried. This time of rest (in prison) has been a great mercy. Everyone here has been very kind. This I would say, standing as I do in view of God and Eternity, I realise that patriotism is not enough. I must have no hatred or bitterness towards anyone.' She asked how she could be sure of going to heaven. Mr Gahan reminded her of the thief on the cross whom Jesus had forgiven with the words, 'Today you shall be with me in Paradise'. 'We shall always remember you as a heroine and as a martyr,' he told her. 'Think of me only as a nurse who tried to do her duty,' she replied.

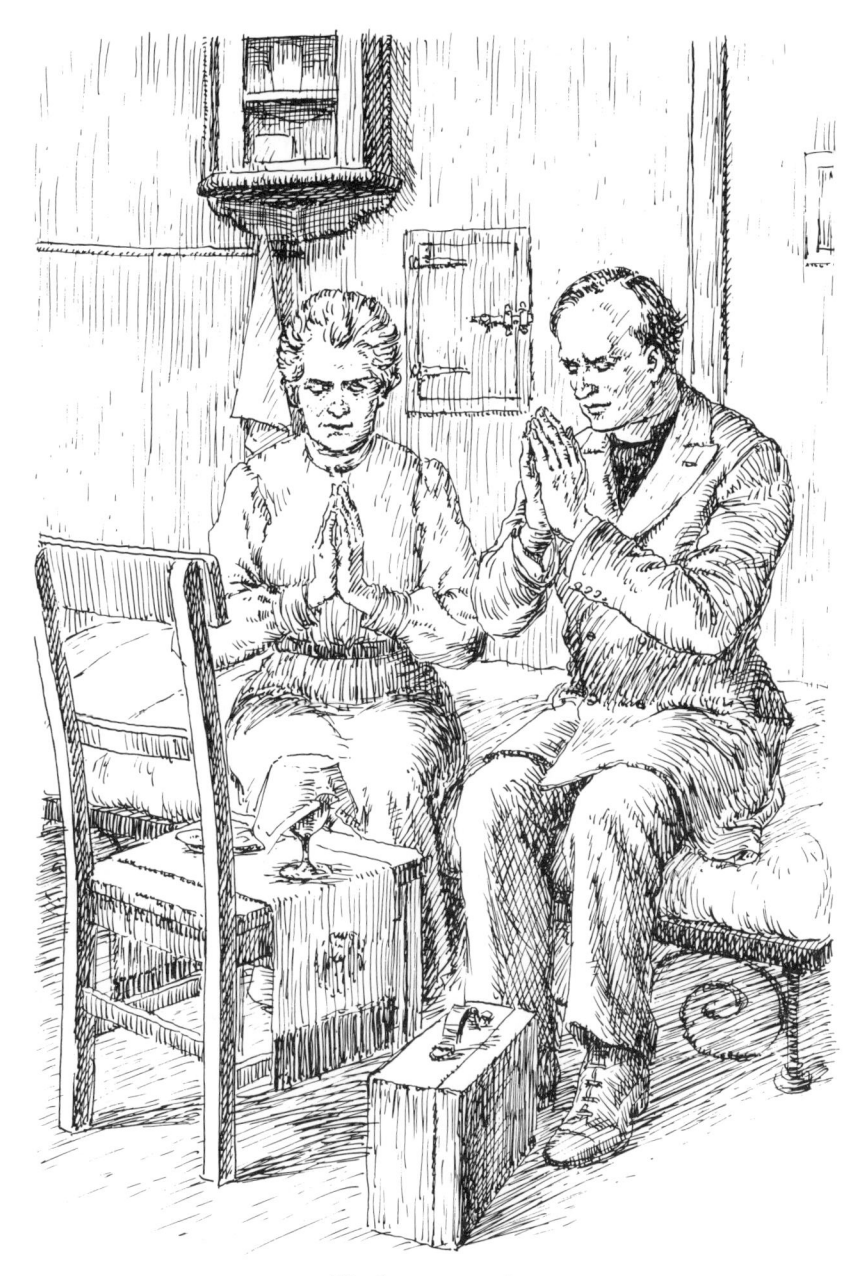

The last communion

After he had gone she wrote to her nurses, urging them to make full use of the new clinic and the opportunities that their work gave them. She begged their forgiveness — 'I have perhaps been unjust sometimes, but I have loved you much more than you think.' She also wrote to her mother.

Several of the nurses were outside the prison when two cars sped out at five o'clock on the morning of Tuesday October 12th. Edith was sitting between two soldiers. Two hundred and fifty more were waiting when she and Philippe Baucq arrived at the national shooting gallery, and were tied to the execution posts. The prison chaplain prayed with her and she said to him, 'Ask Mr Gahan to tell my loved ones that I am glad to die for my country.' There was just time to hand over her little book *The Imitation of Christ*. In it she had written a brief list of the main dates in her life ending: 'Died at 7 a.m. on October 12th 1915. E. Cavell. With love to E. D. Cavell.' It was for her cousin Eddy.

Her eyes were bandaged. Eight soldiers fired. She died at once.

13 The Supreme Lesson

The prison chaplain returned to St Gilles. One of the other prisoners noticed mud on his shoes and a brief conversation took place.
 'You appear already to have gone into the country?'
 'Alas, yes. I accompanied our friends.'
 'Which friends?'
 'Your comrades Philippe Baucq and Miss Cavell.'
 'What . . . . already?'
 'Yes!'
 There was silence.

*   *   *

Back in England the Bishop of Norwich visited Mrs Cavell and found her 'bewildered; her little room was strewn with letters and telegrams.' Her health broke down soon afterwards and she died in 1918 — before Edith's body, which had been hastily buried at the shooting gallery, was brought back to England.
 Other countries bitterly attacked the Germans for Edith's execution. The Germans quickly cancelled the other death sentences. Anger was especially strong in America, where people were already shocked by the way the Germans had sunk the civilian liner *Lusitania* (on which Mme Depage, one of the founders of the clinic, was drowned). The Americans joined Britain in the war in 1917. In England the number of men joining the army doubled almost overnight after Edith died.
 After the war the clinic became known as the Cavell

Institute. All over the world hospital wards, streets and even a mountain peak were named after Edith. In London there is a large statue near Trafalgar Square.

Was Edith's execution fair? Some people have said that although the Germans were very stupid to shoot her, she clearly did help the British war effort, and that she committed treason under German military law. But that law was an unusually harsh one, and her questioning does not seem to have been fair. She was actually executed for taking troops to the enemy — something she did not do herself, and for which no evidence was presented at the trial.

One thing is certain. She was a very brave woman and an excellent Matron. And as the Prime Minister, Mr Asquith, said in 1915: 'She has taught the bravest man among us the supreme lesson of courage.'

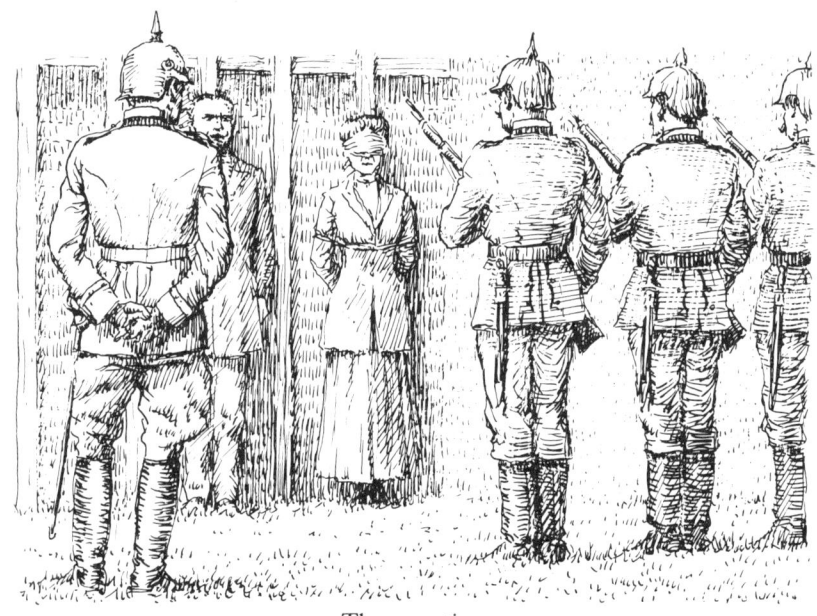

The execution

Important Events in the Life of Edith Cavell (1865-1915)

1865 Born at Swardeston, near Norwich.
1886 Obtains her first job as a children's governess.
1888 Becomes governess to the François family in Belgium.
1895 Returns to England to care for her father.
1896 Begins training as a nurse at the London Hospital.
1907 Returns to Brussels to start the first school for nurses in Belgium.
1912 Appeal started for money for a larger training school.
1914 On holiday in Norfolk when war breaks out. Returns to Brussels. Begins helping Allied soldiers on the run in November.
1915 August 5th: arrested by the Germans
October 7th: trial begins
October 12th: shot at dawn.
1919 Body returned to England and buried outside Norwich Cathedral.

Edith Cavell did not write any books herself, although she described her work in *The Times* and the *Nursing Mirror*. For a fuller description, see *Edith Cavell* by Rowland Ryder, published by Hamish Hamilton in 1975.